CURRENT RESEARCH ON DIETING AND PROVEN WAYS TO MAKE IT WORK FOR LIFE

Anyone Can Lose and Keep It Off

(It's Not That Hard Really)

Presented by Bruce Miller, B.A., J.D.

And

Team Golfwell

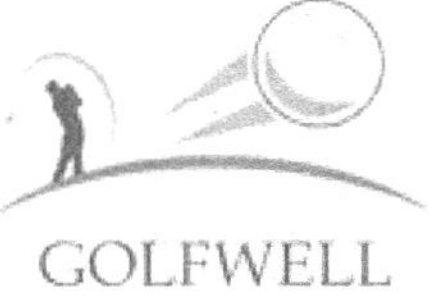

Published by: Pacific Trust Holdings NZ Ltd., 2018

DISCLAIMER. This Book is sold with the understanding that it is a general educational health-related information product and is intended for healthy adults aged 18 and over. We are not physical or mental health medical care providers nor are we nutritionists or dieticians, and the information in this book is not and should not be relied on as professional, psychological, nutritional, or medical advice or treatment.

There may be risks associated with participating in suggestions in this book for people who have a health condition or with pre-existing physical or mental health conditions and you should get a professional medical opinion on whether the information in this book is right for you.

Diets and ways to avoid hunger pangs may be inherently dangerous to certain individuals and can result in medical problems and injury. Do not start any of these suggestions if your physician, nutritionist, or health care provider advises against it. If you suffer any adverse effects, you should seek medical advice immediately.

If you find you still experience hunger pangs after following the suggestions in this book, you should seek immediate medical attention as they may be due to other causes.

While we try to make every effort for the information to be up-to-date and correct, there are no representations or warranties, express or implied, about the completeness, accuracy, reliability, suitability or availability with respect to the information, products, services, or any matter contained in this Book for any purpose. You agree any use of the information in this book is at your own risk.

The publisher and author make no representations with respect to the accuracy or completeness of the contents of this work and specifically disclaim all warranties including without limitation warranties of fitness for a particular purpose. No warranty may be created or extended by promotional or sales materials. The advice and strategies contained herein may not be suitable for every person and/or every situation.

To my daughters, with all my love.

Praises received:

"I found this book seriously helpful since it lets you pick your own diet and gives you documented ways of sticking to it and to keep it off for good.

"I liked the part about having the right state of mind is one key to dieting success. This book brought out that it's no big deal to diet and great success is entirely possible by keeping calm and relaxed about it.

I also liked the research on the variety of ways to eat the right foods, avoid cravings, and many other things. Now I just allow weight loss to happen naturally by following the suggestions in the book. Enjoyed it and it changed my life!"

- Joan Porter

"I especially like the part about using sugar free lozenges to avoid cravings. It works."

- Maria Russo

"A food diary? I hadn't ever used a food journal or a food diary. I do now. I learned about a recent research study that determined people lose 50% more weight if you keep a food diary than if you don't. So, I keep a food diary now and it certainly makes it easier to lose weight. Thank you for doing this book!"

- Clare Peterson

"I could go on and on about this amazing book. Just read it and you'll understand why it's excellent!"

- V. Rosen

"Eating right is now part of my life. This extremely helpful well researched book transformed me! It explains current trends in dieting and the scientific research behind those trends.

Best excerpt, 'Search your inner soul and find the real reason you want to lose weight.'

And, it teaches you how to have a relaxed, calm and lasting healthy attitude toward losing weight and makes it very easy."

- Carol Ann Williamson

"Don't reward yourself by eating crappy food. That's not a reward – it's really giving yourself punishment."

- Drew Carey

Contents

Introduction: Diets Work

Choosing the right food path or diet and sticking to it will result in better health, increased energy, greater self-esteem, and a happier life. This book contains modern research on proven ways to help you do that.

It's also not hard to stick to a diet if you have the right relaxed mental attitude and know how avoid hunger pangs and food cravings. If you know the modern research on current mental attitudes and current ways to avoid hunger pangs and cravings, you will be successful at weight loss and discover losing weight is much easier.

You can adjust your attitude with modern trends and you will be amazed it's not that hard to achieve weight loss and maintain yourself at a healthy lower weight.

The purpose of this book is to show you current scientific research on:

- The right diet mind set

- How to stick to a diet

- How to avoid cravings

- How to deal with hunger pangs

- How to avoid hunger pangs entirely

- How to make it all a lifetime habit.

You will learn:

- How to think healthy

- How to avoid eating unhealthy foods

- Learn new food suggestions

- Learn new eating techniques

- How to easily exercise

- The most popular diets

- And many, many ways to make whatever diet you choose a success.

If you're not on a diet already, first choose a diet which you believe will be successful for you in accordance with the lifestyle you lead. Understand the diet you choose must fit into your lifestyle, i.e., the food in your diet should be readily available to you in your daily routine.

And, get medical advice from your medical advisor on whether the diet you choose is medically suitable for you. Some diets may lead to not having enough of the necessary nutrients you personally require.

Some diets limit your food choices and work for a short term, and any weight you might have lost comes back quick. Try to avoid taking on one of these short-term quick weight loss diets. You should get the best advice from your medical advisor if you have any difficulty in deciding on a diet.

There are many diets to choose from. Popular diets today are the DASH diet, the Mediterranean diet, the Flexitarian Diet, Ketogenic diet, the Atkins diet, the Raw Food diet, the South Beach diet, Weight Watchers, and many others.

Ideally, you want to choose a diet you can live with the rest of your life. Once you have decided on a diet, this book will show you how to incorporate the diet into your life. We discuss how the first 66 days of a diet is the most important time period and how to make it through this period.

There are more than 100 factors or ways to help you make your choice of diet a habit and an integral part of your life in this book.

If you have no trouble sticking to a diet, you don't need to read this book.

But if you do, you should read it.

"I'm totally honest with you. If anyone asks me about how I lost weight, I tell them I have lots of people working on that for me, and I can use Photoshop if nothing else works (Haha)!

"I tell them I can't eat everything I want to eat and still look okay. I was very unhealthy when I was fat, and now I'm just a normal body type. I'm not special; I'm just an actor..."

- Sonam Kapoor

The Right Mental Attitude

On average, scientific researchers have determined it takes a little more than two months (or 66 days on the average) to form a new habit. [1]

In a recent study, researchers found the average time most people needed to form a new habit was 66 days. [2] The researchers also found the time to form a new habit varied between individuals with some only needing less time while others needing more. Overall, the average time to form a new habit was 66 days. [3]

It was previously thought a new habit could be created in 18 to 21 days. This was because plastic surgeons were polled in the 1960s to find out how long it took for women to get used to a new face lift or other cosmetic surgery.

For this book to help you, you first must suggest to yourself you will commit for at least 66 days to the diet you have chosen. It may take you less time or more time to form new eating habits, but once it becomes a habit you have won. We suggest it's best to plan your habit of eating right to become a reality for you in 66 days.

Many psychologists believe when you try to change your eating habits and behavior, it's important to understand it's difficult since we generally believe we have more control over our eating habits than we really do. [4] In addition, our emotions such as stress, worry or addictions to certain foods conflict with our logical minds and we tend to rationalize and go off the diet. [5]

Our genes, heredity, emotions, and habits are all interacting at the same time when we make food decisions. Even though heredity may contribute to you being overweight, you need to keep in mind that kind of thinking (i.e., blaming it on heredity) will demotivate you on your journey to have a healthy weight for yourself.

To avoid stress, a positive attitude toward a diet in a relaxed manner will usually make you succeed with your weight loss goals. Susan McQuillan, M.S. RDN wrote an interesting article on this in Psychology Today showing it really isn't hard if you relax and put your wellbeing first and just let it happen. [6]

Emma Seppala, Ph.D., the Science Director of Stanford University's Center for Compassion and Altruism Research and Education, in her book, "The Happiness Track," said we are better people when we relax and put our own wellbeing first. She found that we sometimes think we need to put off our happiness to become successful. She pointed out if you look at the data, when you relax and make your wellbeing your first priority, the data suggests you will actually be more successful and performing better as well as have better relationships…" [7]

The National Weight Loss Registry keeps track of people who have successfully lost weight and kept it off for many years. [8]

The National Weight Loss Registry keeps records on thousands of people who have lost significant amounts of weight. These people have kept the weight they lost off for more than a year and many up to five years or more (about 60 lbs. on average). The NWLR follows up and updates their records on the people who register with them.

If you are over 18 years old and have lost weight and kept it off, you may want to look into becoming part of their research. See their website. [9] You may want to become part of their study and the National Weight Loss people will provide you with additional support in attaining your weight loss goals. [10]

Find your main motivation for weight loss:

Search your inner soul and find the real reason you desire to lose weight.

This is one of the most important things to do to be successful at whatever diet you choose to follow.

To achieve success with your diet (again check with your medical advisor before beginning any weight loss plan), look deeply into yourself to try and understand and recognize *exactly why* you want to lose weight. It can be a positive reason, e.g. to fit into a wedding dress.

For men, some may want to lose weight for more body definition, so they don't mind it when they take their shirt off.

Or, your main reason may be for better health, or a healthier heart, and it's best to pick a specific health reason you can focus us (rather than a general reason) for wanting to lose weight, etc.

Your main reason for going on a diet can also be a negative reason, e.g. sick of being embarrassed and awkward, can't afford to buy larger clothes, your significant other may be drifting away from you, etc.

If you have a loved one or trusted friend who will keep whatever you say confidential, discuss it with that person and try to identify your exact reason(s) for weight loss.

If you identify in your soul the exact reason(s) you want to lose weight, this will give you an unstoppable and a very strong motivation to succeed and you will reach your goals. You need to know your innermost feelings and disregard superficial reasons. In other words, get in touch with and understand your main reason(s) on why you want to lose weight. Meditate, discuss it with a trusted friend or loved one, and think deeply to discover what your foremost reason is for your weight loss desires.

Find one reason to focus on but you may have two or more equally heartfelt reasons to lose weight. After you identify your innermost reason(s) for deciding to lose weight, use that reason(s) as your focus and obsession. This will help you avoid rationalization, so you won't be telling yourself it's okay to give into a craving just this one time.

Celebrate your small and large victories. As you begin or maintain your diet and successfully overcome cravings, internally celebrate your victories with yourself for making good food choices so it's felt deep in your heart.

For example, if you turn down desert, or eat smaller portions, or conquer a craving, etc., then you should pause, feel it and remember it deep in your heart. If you carry a small victory journal, write each victory down and tell yourself you are succeeding.

Whether you know it or not, each small victory will automatically lead to more success and gradually build your confidence on your journey to a new body. In other words, the more you appreciate each small victory, the easier it becomes to continue.

This is because research scientists have proven success breeds more success. [11] Each time you succeed in any small way, you should briefly pause, feel proud and happy. By doing so you are making it easier for yourself to continue to succeed in turning down deserts, taking smaller portions, etc. in the future.

For even more mental strength, ask your loved ones and those who love you for their emotional support to help you establish new habits over the next 66 days. Emotional support [12] of loved ones and a good friend are proven major factors in helping you to change your behavior and develop new habits during the next 66 days. A diet buddy is also very helpful to contribute to your support to change eating habits.

At the same time, avoid (or spend the least amount of time with) people who don't support you on your journey to develop new habits. If you cannot avoid them, change the subject if the conversation turns to anything involving weight loss or food.

Also, you can get additional support by joining a local weight loss club, a Weight Watcher group, or Weight Loss Meetup Groups.

To keep a positive attitude, recognize any negative thoughts which might pop up in your brain about your dieting and dismiss those thoughts immediately or as fast as you can. Avoid thinking about the difficulties in losing weight. This is because thinking about the tribulations of dieting creates anxiety and you need to stay calm and relaxed about it. And, the more you think about dieting, the more you may overthink and exaggerate the task ahead, especially if you haven't succeeded in dieting before.

Remember, simply being on a diet is far better than taking no action at all. [13] Thinking and worrying about the dieting process of losing weight doesn't help you one bit. And, forget about any feelings of worry, nervousness, anticipated hunger pangs, irritability, feelings of failure, etc. Simply get into it and do it in a relaxed manner and sincerely applaud every success you have turning down desserts, etc. for the next 66 days.

Take it only one day at a time for the first 66 days. After that, your personal eating habits will be an integral part of a happier and healthier you. Keep reminding yourself of your innermost heart felt reason(s) for changing your eating habits over the next 66 days. Be calm and confident about it reminding yourself of your innermost and upmost reason(s) for losing weight. This will help you keep mentally strong.

To further strengthen your resolve, write out the reason(s) on an index card on why you sincerely want to change your eating habits and refer to it often.

Remember what you looked like when you were not overweight? Form a picture of your previous self in your mind and think about what your looked like before you became overweight. Keep that positive picture of yourself before you were overweight in your mind. If you have an actual picture of your old self, keep it handy on your phone to inspire you for the next 66 days.

Likewise, keep a negative mental picture of your overweight self. You should find yourself becoming determined not to ever be overweight again. This will help you fight off cravings or desserts. Remind yourself and continually reaffirm to yourself, you don't want to be or look overweight ever again.

Before eating anything, pause and visualize in your mind a picture of yourself being thin again. Visualize yourself with an increase in energy, agility and a better looking and healthier you. Positively thinking of yourself reaching the ideal weight range you seek to enjoy will help you establish new eating habits.

Train your mind to flash an alert if you find yourself sinking back into old eating habits during the first 66 days. Allow a very bright light bulb to flash and a siren to go off in your mind in case you find yourself acquiescing to your old ways.

When you find yourself falling into an old eating habits, pause and stop yourself by positively visualizing yourself in the weight range you want to be in.

Be patient and go slow and remember you will increase your ability to disregard old eating habits with each success you have when you refuse to eat the way you used to. This will lead you to more successes as the days and weeks go by in the first 66 days. [14]

For whatever reason(s), if you think there might be a good chance of you not reaching your ideal weight range, set a very high weight loss goal. If you don't reach your very high weight loss goal, you won't feel exasperated in not reaching your very high goal, but you will feel like a winner if you only reach a percentage of the very high goal.

When you are on your relaxed journey to get back to your ideal weight, set small goals for yourself which will give you more positive victories as you reach each small goal. You will be more reinforced when you reach and enjoy each small goal you set for yourself.

Set a hundred or more goals for yourself during the next 66 days and it is important to celebrate as you reach each one. For example, keep track of how many desserts you turned down, how many times you ate a smaller portion, how many good food choices you made, how many times you turned down old food choices, how many times you exercised, how many times you didn't eat past 7 pm in the evening, how many times your thinking changed when you disregarded old choices or didn't even think of food, etc.

Consider rewarding yourself with something (other than food) for every success you achieve. For example, if you feel you accomplished a large goal or milestone marker in your weight loss journey, see a great movie, sell old clothes which are too big on eBay or donate them charity, get a massage or a facial, schedule a gym session with a friend or a personal trainer, get new shoes, etc.

If you play sports, experience and rejoice how easier it is to play your favorite sport with less weight.

Most importantly, tell yourself you are doing it and you are succeeding at it, and you will reach your goal(s). Remember to smile more than you usually do.

To help your mind leave old habits behind you, remember the adage, "Out of sight is out of mind" and eliminate all unhealthy treats or other unhelpful foods from your residence. Only shop grocery stores with a pre-written list so you don't supply yourself with anything that will be harmful for you during the next 66 days. Go around point of sale locations in grocery stores quickly and don't be distracted by low prices or items you don't need.

If you are going to a party, a dinner, or other social event where there will be unhelpful or unhealthy sugary foods, eat helpful foods *before* you go so you will not eat as much or at least eat smaller portions while attending. If remarks are made on how little you eat, turn the conversation away from yourself and away from food. Ask non-food related questions (hobbies, children, etc.) to others and get people talking about themselves (most people love to talk about themselves anyway). Order small healthy protein dishes at restaurants.

Eat at home more than usual during the next 66 days which will help you get your mind on things other than food and you'll save money as well.

To avoid eating unhealthy sugary food, sincerely consider, pause and reflect on the long-term effect. If you realize and understand one donut will keep you where you don't want to be, that is a victory in your thinking and such a victory will increase your mental strength on future food choices making it easier each time you make a good choice.

Be aware and understand by delaying instant gratification, you will become closer to forming new eating habits. You want to have the number of your daily calories you expend exceed the number of calories you ingest.

If you carry a lunch to your job, use a paper bag or an opaque lunch box rather than a clear container you can see through.

Keep a patient attitude. Understand today's instant gratification society with texting, Skype, Snapchat, Personal Data Assistants, etc. all tend to make a person think that things can be done very quickly. Weight loss takes a calm, relaxed and patient attitude. Don't be in a rush to lose weight. It will happen.

Some medical experts recommend a weight loss program resulting in 1-2 lbs. per week (depending on your present weight, of course). [15]

In a gym, a popular attitude is "no pain, no gain" making you think you must suffer to reach the goals you set in your weight loss program. However, you should approach weight loss in an easy and relaxed manner. "No pain, no gain" is not a good attitude. Weight loss and weight management is not that hard if you are patient.

Have a healthy attitude confirming to yourself you have made a commitment and you are going to try and stick with it. Avoid any negative thoughts where you feel you really can't do it.

An excellent way to remove a negative attitude is not to compare yourself with others. Or, if you tend to compare yourself with others and run into people who have lost weight and kept it off, think to yourself, "*I can do it too.*" And keep reaffirming that attitude of "I can do it" to yourself.

Be mindful, everyone is different and eating habits for some people may not be right for you. The brain takes time to communicate a fullness feeling (you should allow at least 15 to 20 minutes for the brain to catch up to what you just ate). You will read more about this 15 to 20-minute delay later in this book.

Have a mental image of yourself as a new person enjoying the weight range you desire. If you find yourself falling back to old eating habits, tell yourself you are not that person anymore. Tell yourself you are in a new wonderful lifestyle now which doesn't include the self-indulgent consumption of high calorie food and overeating. Tell yourself you are headed for a wonderful life as you reach each goal as you leave your old self behind and welcome the changes which will happen to your physique.

Tell yourself once you've lost the weight to reach your goal(s) you are not going to go back and fall into the overeating lifestyle which was embarrassing and destructive to your self-esteem and confidence.

Don't let yourself become disappointed with the slow process of weight loss. Understand being on a diet normally will make you lose weight during the first weeks and weight loss becomes slower as you come closer to your goal.

Feel happy that your weight loss might be slowing down since this means you are getting closer to your goal and soon you will have achieved what you always wanted. Look forward to living with and enjoying a thinner, lighter and more agile physique.

Weigh yourself once a week. If you get tired or bored by weighing yourself, measure your Body Mass Index (BMI). There are several sites on the web which will compute your BMI for you. [16]

Keep in mind when you weigh yourself, your weight will fluctuate as you gradually lose weight. Your weight may even increase even though you are sticking to your diet. Understand increases in weight can be the result from various other causes so don't get discouraged. If you consume salt, your body may retain water which adds to your weight and body definition so limit salt if you can.

Keep in mind the main reason most people gain weight (and keep the weight on) is they consume more calories than they expend. Be aware of this principle and adjust your exercise and food intake accordingly so that you will be expending more calories than you consume each day.

Remind yourself you aren't going to return to the pattern of your old ways. If you do, realize you will regain the weight back that you had when you started, or perhaps even more weight as you age.

Breaking bad habits (like eating sugary foods, overeating or smoking) take about the same time as it takes to form new habits. [17] So, be patient, relaxed and calm about it.

Proven Ways to Make It Work For Life

Researchers at Nature Neuroscience did a 15-year study trying to find out what part of the human brain controls cravings. They determined cravings were caused by a certain area of neurons in the brain which are responsible for hunger and feeling full (satiety). [18]

They researched this area of the brain and drew an interesting conclusion on why most people seem to regain the weight they lost when they were on a diet. They found the lost weight is regained since after a person loses 5% to 10% of body weight, these neurons become active causing feelings of hunger. In other words, the body senses a smaller amount of calories are being consumed daily than what the body previously consumed and consequently activate those neurons and other parts of the body to make a person crave food most of the time. [19] The researchers felt this was the major reason why most diets fail even though a person lost weight initially. [20]

However, their research has also showed the mind will eventually adjust to your new weight so that you will not feel hungry most of the time. Research is continuing in this area to determine the exact nature of food cravings and feelings of hunger and satiety. Perhaps someday after you lose weight the researchers might come up with a pill you could take to make you feel full until it is time to eat again.

Many people have successfully overcome cravings for unhealthy food on their own without a miracle pill. Jonathan Bricker, Ph.D. gave a lecture recorded on a very popular 15-minute YouTube video named "The Secret to Self-Control". [21] This YouTube (which has had over 3 million views) shows you how to train your brain to eat less and ways to deal with cravings and not have them bother you and go away forever.

Jonathan Bricker suggests we put a pause or a beat in our thought process when we experience cravings for food (he discusses cravings for tobacco as well on the video). The brief pause or beat in our thoughts gives our brain time to think instead of coaxing you to get instant gratification, i.e. eat food.

Dr. Bricker suggests a person should pause and recognize the craving and think about it for a moment and this pause routine will lessen the craving and make it go away.

There are other ways to distract your thinking away from unhealthy food such as making a list you can refer to instantly for activities you could do when you experience a craving. Some of these activities might be:

- Brush your teeth since most people don't feel like eating after they've brushed their teeth.

- Put a sugar free lozenge in your mouth to slowly dissolve.

- You may be thirsty instead of hungry so drink water and see how you feel after 8 oz to 16 oz of water (more on drinking water later in this book).

- Do an exercise video, or do 50 toe touches, or 20 pushups, etc.

- Walk around the block.

- Play a video game.

- Walk your dog.

- Polish your nails.

- Add as many activities to your list as you can and keep it handy when you first go on a diet.

If you experience stress, performing exercises reduces stress. So, if you experience cravings, pause and take time out for exercise.

For example, the massive Fitness Blender [22] website offers hundreds of free exercise videos including low impact workouts, beginner workouts, simple stretching exercises, Core Exercises, advanced HIIT (High Intensity Interval Training) workouts, insane workouts to exhaust yourself, etc.

The Fitness Blender exercise videos range from videos which are only a few minutes long to over 80 minute videos. They provide a wide and varied selection of exercise videos to fit most everyone – there's even an exercise video for people who get bored easily.

Exercise will not only relieve stress and tension, but also begin to reshape your body.

If you like sports, spend more time doing the sports you like and that will clear your head as well. Swimming, tennis, dancing, or any sport you like usually leads to a reduction of stress and anxiety as well as help you expend calories and lose weight. Pick an activity you truly enjoy and mix it up with other activities to avoid boredom.

All of this will strengthen your resolve and make it easier for you to form a new habit of healthy ways to avoid cravings which will lead you to a very healthy and happy life.

Another way to avoid cravings is to make sure you eat regularly and don't go more than 4 hours without eating. Not eating can lead to an increased appetite which makes most people overeat.

When you eat a smaller portion, try using a smaller plate and eat it slowly. If you've been eating every 4 hours, you shouldn't find yourself being overly hungry with a voracious appetite causing you to overeat. Take your time, study the food, feel its texture when you put it in your mouth and chew the food at least 20 – 40 times in your mouth.

If you are a person whose nature it is to always be on a "Seefood" diet, i.e. you "see food and compulsively eat it" - or what some people call a "spontaneous eater," schedule motivational quotes on your phone every half hour or hour to remind yourself not to overeat. Here are just a few:

- "Nothing tastes as good as being fit feels."

- "Eat to nourish your body, not to feed your emotions."

- "Losing weight might be difficult but being overweight is a much more difficult way to go through life."

- "Unhealthy sugary foods make your clothes shrink."

- "Your body is what you carry through life. The more it weighs the shorter it will be."

- "I'm on the "Quit Eating Crap Food Diet."

- "Don't give up what you want most for a fleeting moment's pleasure."

- "If I spent the time I spend thinking about unhealthy and sugary food and used that time to exercise instead, I would look like a supermodel."

- "The only bad exercise sessions are the sessions you didn't do."

- "If I ever get tired of starting a diet repeatedly, I am telling myself right now not to give up this time and just calmly get through it and form good habits. Now is the right time to finally get this done."

- "I'm not on a diet, I'm changing and improving my life to much better things."

- "You must believe in yourself even when no one else does and if you can do that, you are already a winner." - Venus Williams

- "I am focusing on what my new life will be like with my new body."

- A protein shake toast: "Let's raise a glass to better habits, better life, better eating, better health, and loving ourselves."

- "When you want to give up, remember and reflect on your deepest reason(s) on losing weight."

- "Your diet is like money in your bank. Excellent choices of food are great investments." - Bethanny Frankel

- "People have to realize that dieting is a marathon. Take your time and celebrate every small victory and you will win the race." - Ian K. Smith

- Don't let one bad day become three bad days.

- They really need to take the "s" out of fast food.

- "Stomach, I think you are just bored and not hungry so shut up."

- One or more bad decisions won't stop you from your goal. Nothing will stop you.

- Be proud and applaud yourself with every small victory along the way.

- I am determined to do all things which will make the rest of my life - the very best of my life.

- I have a new vision of myself that makes me jump out of bed every morning.

The above are just a few quotes. Add your own inspirational and motivational quotes as reminders to help you adjust during the first few days and to keep them going for 66 days.

There are also free Inspirational Quote Apps on the web such as Motivate: Daily Motivation [23] and many others you can put on your phone.

Dr. Howard LeWine, M.D., and Chief Medical Editor of Harvard Health Publishing recommended not eating anything while watching TV or doing anything distracting. [24] He said, "You will eat more if you are watching TV, the computer screen, or any kind of multitasking when you are eating something." [25]

If you find you lose concentration because of hunger pangs, cravings, delicious food aromas (delicious food aromas cause hormones to be released which aggravate the cravings), sip a protein shake. It will suppress the cravings and make you feel satiated. According to the Society for Endocrinology, when you consume protein, a hormone is released called Peptide YY which makes you feel full and satisfied. [26]

More Proven Ways for Effective Eating

Restaurant Menus. In September 2018, researchers at Cornell University studied a restaurant (which was a full-service restaurant) that posted the calorie content next to each menu item. The restaurant also had a menu which didn't show calories. The patrons who used the menu with the calories shown ate 45 calories less on average than the other group who ordered off the menu which didn't show the calorie content.

An interesting finding was that the patrons with the calories shown ordered less calorie food in appetizer and main dish sections, but both groups ordered approximately the same calories when it came to desserts and drinks. [27]

Breakfast. If you are on a low carb diet, you may not be hungry when you get up in the morning. Nevertheless, you should eat breakfast to prevent later cravings in the morning and prevent snacking between breakfast and lunch. Also, skipping breakfast lowers your blood sugar and increases your appetite so you will eat more at your next meal.

Water. Keep yourself fully hydrated and drink at least eight glasses of water per day.

You might mistake feelings of being thirsty for food cravings. This is because a scientific study showed that it is very easy to mistake being hungry for being thirsty. This study known as "Relationships Between Human Thirst, Hunger, Drinking, and Feeding" and was published by the National Center for Biotechnology Information (NCBI). This study found people mistook being hungry for being thirsty. People incorrectly ate food instead of drinking water and this occurs at least 60% of the time. [28]

In other words, people mistook being thirsty for hunger most of the time. This is because there is an area in your brain called the hypothalamus which controls both hunger and thirst, and researchers found the hunger and thirst signals get crossed 60% of the time. [29]

If you feel hungry, drink water instead of eating and wait 15 - 20 minutes for your brain to process the water to see if you were thirsty or hungry. Some people love good food, or they may worry they have not had enough to eat, or they may have slow metabolisms and continue to eat before their brain catches up to signals in their body that they've consumed enough food. If you feel you are that type of person, make a mental note of the time you stop eating when you finished your dinner. Wait 15-20 minutes and see if you still feel like eating more.

Also, many studies have shown people who drank 16 oz. of water before eating ate less than people who didn't drink water before eating. The people who drank water on average consumed about 75 less calories. [30]

Protein drinks. If you sip a protein drink (or water) while dieting, the liquid (especially the protein drink) should quiet hunger pangs as well as keep you hydrated.

Low Cal Soup and Liquids. Studies have been done to show consuming low-calorie soup and low-calorie liquids before eating will reduce your appetite.

Sugar. Avoid sugary food or treats that have corn syrup, glucose, high-fructose corn syrup, brown sugar, honey, maltose, corn sweeteners and dextrose. Many studies have been done which show foods with these types of ingredients make it difficult to control your appetite and you will wind up eating more than you need to eat.

Snacks. According to the Mayo Clinic Staff, snacks between meals should be limited to an item with less than 100 calories. [31]

Slow. Remember to eat slowly. Several studies have found eating slowly allows you to feel satiated faster than if you eat fast. Harvard Health reports a lot of research which has shown it takes 15 - 20 minutes for the brain to recognize you have eaten enough food. Allow the chemistry to be processed by your brain so your brain can catch up with your eating. [32]

One way to slow down your eating style is to put smaller portions on your fork and chew slowly at least 20 times per forkful.

Multitasking while eating. Prof. Jeff Brunstrom, an experimental psychologist at the Univ. of Liverpool performed an experiment on whether eating with a distraction inhibits memory encoding for a meal, which, would in turn, increase later food intake.

In one experiment, his subjects were asked to eat while playing a solitaire video game. Another group of subjects ate the same amount of food without any distractions. Those that played the game snacked *much* more before their next meal than the subjects who weren't distracted. [33] In other words, Dr. Brunstrom found when you are distracted you forget how much you've eaten which makes you eat more until your next meal. More on remembering what you've eaten last later in this book to help you avoid cravings.

Chew gum. Studies have shown chewing sugarless – low calorie gum before and after meals reduced both appetite and hunger. If your appetite is reduced, you will eat less and consume less calories. Try to chew gum (if you like gum) before eating and you should wind up taking smaller portions.

High Fiber foods. High fiber foods like beans, grains, celery, peas, lentils, etc. will make you feel fuller. One science study has researched viscous fibers which contain glucomannan which are believed to reduce appetite. [34] These fibers are high in vitamins, minerals, and other healthful nutrients. It was found fibers which are more viscous which contain glucomannan such as beans (legumes), flax seeds, asparagus, brussels sprouts, oats, etc. reduce appetite. [35]

Solid v. Liquid Calories. Calories from solid foods will give you more of a feeling of fullness than calories from liquids. Solid calories will decrease your appetite more than liquid calories. This is because when you consume solid foods, it takes more time to chew the food than drinking a liquid. The additional time involved in consuming solid foods gives your brain more time to feel full. *Coffee.* Caffeinated or decaffeinated coffee, like protein, causes the release of peptide YY, which will decrease your appetite and promote a feeling of being full.

Use a big fork. The New York Times reported a research study was done to see if people ate less when they ate with a bigger fork.

The study found people ate more when they used a smaller fork since they thought they weren't putting enough food in their mouths with a smaller fork and consequently ate more. So, if you use a larger fork, you will eat less than what you would eat using a smaller fork. [36]

Sleep. Researchers have found if you don't get enough sleep you will eat more than you do when you get 7-8 hours' sleep per night. [37] This is because you have less mental sharpness and will power when you don't get enough sleep. [38]

Avoid stressful eating. Many studies have found people who are stressed tend to eat more than when they are not stressed although some of the subjects lost their appetite when stressed. One study found 81% of people change their eating habits when stressed. Of this 81%, 62 % ate more food when stressed and 38% ate nothing or less than what they normally eat. [39]

Omega-3 Fats. Foods with Omega-3 fats, (like salmon, tuna, sardines, i.e., cold water fish) increase feelings of fullness in overweight people.

Remember your last meal. Psychologist, Eric Robinson, Ph.D. of the Institute of Psychology Health and Society, University of Liverpool, has written an article where he found a person does not eat as much if at the time he sits down for his next meal, he pauses and recalls what he ate at his last meal. Remembering what you had to eat last will reduce hunger pangs as well. [40]

Remembering portions. Professor Jeff Brunstrom at the University of Bristol had students eat a bowl of soup. Some of them were eating out of a small bowl which had a special feature which allowed the small bowl to be topped up without the student realizing it. It was done by a tube through the table which refilled the small bowl.

The other group of students ate from a much larger and non-refillable bowl.

Because of the refilling, the students who ate from the smaller bowl ate more than the students with the larger bowl.

Prof. Brunstrom studied the later snacking of both groups and found that those who thought they consumed more soup from a larger bowl snacked less than those who ate out of a smaller bowl. The smaller bowl students (who ate more) snacked more than the students who ate a lot less soup out of a larger bowl. [41] In other words, those who *thought* they ate more snacked less.

You should reflect on your last meal before snacking or eating your next meal. If you had a large meal, remember and pause and reflect on that large meal to avoid snacking and overeating at your next meal.

There have been experiments on distracted eating which make people forget what they've eaten, as reported in a research paper entitled, "Television and eating: repetition enhances food intake." It has been researched many times and people do in fact ingest more food when distracted. [42] Distractions make people forget how much they've eaten and it's important to remember how much food you've taken in.

Skip meals? We discussed not skipping breakfast before especially if you are on a low carb diet. This is because skipping any meal may lead to increased hunger which will lead to overeating. If you need to plan a schedule for your meals. Some people prefer 3 meals a day, while other prefer 5 or 6 very small meals per day. No matter what your schedule, try not to skip a meal.

Exercise. It has become well established that exercise will not make you hungrier. Exercise will actually reduce your hunger. [43] So, try exercise to reduce cravings or hunger pangs. Do a quick jog or some form of exercise for 15 minutes when you have a craving or have hunger pangs when you have eaten enough already.

Out of sight – Out of mind. Studies have shown you won't be tempted in stores which get rid of candy bars near checkouts. [44] Dr. Deborah Cohen in her article on the Rand Blog, "Out of Sight, Out of Mind" explains if you get rid of unhealthy foods such as candy bars, donuts, candies, etc. from your sight you will think of them less. [45] Remove all of them from your residence, workplace, etc.

Raw Fruits & Veggies. Raw fruit and vegetables contain fiber which keep you feeling fuller for longer periods. Fiber from fruits and veggies are an excellent way to feel fuller longer rather than eating other foods. When you feel fuller, you eat less.

Losing belly fat. Fat around the midsection is linked strongly to heart disease and other diseases and there is a lot of material written about how to lose it. It is difficult to sift through the massive amounts of information to find a genuine way to lose belly fat.

However, Kris Gunnars has written an excellent article, in our opinion, on 6 effective ways to specifically lose belly fat. [46]

More Proven Ways: Foods That Minimize Hunger Pangs

The Satiety Index List. [47] Some foods make you feel fuller than others. That is, they have a higher satiety value. Check the foods in the following satiety index list to see if any of the most filling foods are in your present diet. [48]

To compare one against another food, white bread is given of reference and set value of 100%.

The following satiety list shows common foods *by category* which make you feel more or less full than if you ate the same amount of white bread. That is, if the food has a value over 100%, eating that food will make you feel fuller than if you ate the same amount of white bread. If the food has a value less than 100% it will make you feel *less* full than if you ate the same amount of white bread.

Here are the satiety values for common foods by category:

Bakery Products

Croissant 47%

Cake 65%

Doughnuts 68%

Cookies 120%

Crackers 127%

Snacks and Confectionary

Mars candy bar 70%

Peanuts 84%

Yogurt 88%

Crisps 91%

Ice cream 96%

Jellybeans 118%

Popcorn 154%

All-Bran 151%

Porridge/Oatmeal 209%

Breakfast Cereals with Milk

Muesli 100%

Sustain 112%

Special K 116%

Cornflakes 118%

Honeysmacks 132%

Carbohydrate-Rich Foods

White bread 100%

French fries 116%

White pasta 119%

Brown Rice 132%

White rice 138%

Grain bread 154%

Whole meal bread 157%

Brown pasta 188%

Potatoes boiled 323%

Protein-Rich Foods

Lentils 133%

Cheese 146%

Eggs 150%

Baked beans 168%

Beef 176%

Ling fish 225%

Fruits

Bananas 118%

Grapes 162%

Oranges 202%

Apples 197%

The above list shows common foods *per category*. Here is the list again with the most filling common foods listed first.

Potatoes boiled 323%

Ling fish 225%

Porridge/Oatmeal 209%

Oranges 202%

Apples 197%

Brown pasta 188%

Beef 176%

Baked beans 168%

Grapes 162%

Whole meal bread 157%

Grain bread 154%

Popcorn 154%

Eggs 150%

Cheese 146%

White rice 138%

Lentils 133%

Brown Rice 132%

Honeysmacks 132%

All-Bran 151%

Crackers 127%

Cookies 120%

White pasta 119%

Bananas 118%

Jellybeans 118%

Cornflakes 118%

Special K 116%

French fries 116%

White bread 100%

Muesli 100%

Ice cream 96%

Crisps 91%

Yogurt 88%

Peanuts 84%

Mars candy bar 70%

Doughnuts 68%

Cake 65%

Croissant 47%

The Satiety value was started by an Australian doctor, Susanna Holt in 1995. The foods which have a high value stay in your stomach longer than those foods with a less value.

More foods that make you feel fuller. Beginning with eggs, the following describe different foods which make you feel full. These foods are usually included in most diets. If they are not included in your diet, consider adding these foods as an additional way to feel fuller if these foods would fit well with the diet you've chosen. These more filling foods will help you stay on your diet.

Eggs. Eggs are protein which are very satisfying and make you feel fuller for longer than many other foods. Not only do you feel fuller, but eggs also help prevent you from overeating at your next meal.

The Austrian Tribune reported a scientific study showing eating eggs help you to stay fit. [49] Eggs clearly reduced hunger. One experiment involved two groups where the first group had eggs for breakfast and the other group had cereal. To test the subsequent hunger of each group, a lunch was given to the groups three hours later. The group that had eggs ate much less than the other group. [50]

Dietician Dr. Carrie Ruxton who studied the report said, "Eggs are nature's appetite suppressant and consuming eggs leads to eating less at the next meal." [51]

The Tribune reported this is first time research which revealed hormone levels involving the hormone PYY – a satiety hormone which increases when you eat eggs making you feel fuller. [52]

Oats. Oats have a high satiety value and are low in calories but are higher in carbs. Oats contain fiber which slows digestion.

Legumes. Beans, peas, lentils are fibrous and have a high satiety value and contain vegetable protein.

Cottage Cheese. Cottage cheese has a high satiety value and is low in carbs and high in protein.

Quinoa. This grain is high in protein and is digested slowly and has a high satiety value.

Boiled Potatoes. Boiled potatoes have one of the highest satiety food values. It has more carbohydrates than you may be aware of if you are trying a low carb diet. Potatoes strongly curb appetites.

Fish. Fish have a higher satiety value than chicken or eggs and fish like salmon have healthy Omega – 3 fatty acids.

Almonds. Almonds have a high satiety value since they contain fat which cuts off hunger pangs more than other foods. A handful of Almonds is a filling snack if you eat them when you are not distracted, and you eat them slowly. After eating a handful wait 15-20 minutes before eating any more to allow your brain to tell you feel full. If you don't wait those minutes, you may find yourself munching more almonds down when your brain will soon be telling you that you already have had enough.

Also, several studies show chewing almonds slowly (up to 40 times) before swallowing made people less hungry. [53]

Tea. Like coffee and decaffeinated coffee, tea will suppress hunger pangs.

Oranges and Grapefruit. Both fruits will help you defeat cravings and hunger pangs as both are high in fiber and have a high satiety value.

Good Fats like Avocados. When you eat good fats, a hormone named leptin is released from the fat inside your body. According to Web MD if you eat only a small amount of fats, only a small amount of leptin is released which increases your appetite. [54] A larger amount of leptin will decrease your appetite. And, conversely, a lack of leptin causes a high appetite whether you need the food or not.

Soybeans or Soy. Soybeans contain fat, protein and carbohydrates. They curb hunger and keep your appetite in control.

Nuts. Nuts likewise have protein and fiber and control appetite since nuts (especially almonds) are high in healthy (monounsaturated) fats. Healthy fats are good to help you lose weight, prevent the risk of heart disease, and other benefits. For example, try eating a few almonds (or a small amount of tuna or chicken) with high fiber vegetables like peas and drink 12 oz. of water and you won't have any cravings for at least 3 hours.

Drinking 12 oz. of water with high fiber foods helps the undigested fiber in your stomach expand to make you feel fuller much longer.

Protein. When you eat protein, you feel satisfied longer since protein causes your body to release appetite suppressing hormones. Drinking a small cup of whey protein will make you eat less and consume less calories before eating a meal.

Spicy foods. The NCBI reported that Capsaicin which is found in red chili peppers will help you lose weight. The report explains several Capsaicin experiments where people ate less when they added it (i.e. through adding chili powder or pepper) to their food and helpful in dealing with obesity. [55]

Green tea. Green tea burns fat and suppresses your appetite since your body treats green tea as an appetite suppressant like protein does. It also fights obesity, type II diabetes and is good for your heart. [56]

Artificial Sweeteners. Harvard Health Publishing reports that the body reactions to artificial sweeteners is complex and they may even cause you to overeat. [57] Dr. David Ludwig, a Bariatric Physician, at a Harvard affiliated hospital has stated his concerns whether artificial sweeteners have too many harmful effects and may lead to gaining more weight. He explained people knowingly or unknowingly "fool themselves" by thinking if they drink a diet soda, then they have the right to an extra-large fries and wind up eating more. [58]

Dietary fats. The Nutrition Journal of Bio Med Central reported there are healthy items of plant and seafood which have good monounsaturated and polyunsaturated fats and are important to your diet." [59] Avocados, salmon and other foods contain healthy fats which are beneficial and help you to avoid food with unhealthy fats found in highly processed snack food. [60]

High Quality and Portions. According to the Harvard School of Public Health, the best overall diet is a balanced diet with high quality (not processed) foods in proper portions for a lifetime of good health. [61] For a weight loss plan, they reported there isn't a "one size fits all diet" due to differences in lifestyles (as far as they know).

The Harvard School of Public Health recommends unrefined foods such as vegetables and fruits, whole grains, healthy fats and healthy sources of protein. There is a list of these foods in their Healthy Eating Plate. [62]

More Proven Ways: When All Else Fails

If you diligently follow your diet and stay within the rules of your diets but don't lose weight, seek medical advice from your health professional.

If your doctor says you are healthy, the following are other ways to lose weight and avoid cravings and hunger pangs.

Do pushups. Doing pushups will increase heart rate and burn calories. Doing pushups can also mean doing "pushups from the dinner table." In other words, use sheer will power and determination to eat smaller portions and get yourself away from the dinner table.

Fasting (Intermittent Fasting). One method of fasting is the 16 - 8 - hour method. An example of this method of fasting would be if you finish eating for the day at say 7pm. You then fast for 16 hours. You don't eat anything until 16 hours later or 11am the next day. Then you eat 2 or 3 normal meals of healthy food within the next 8 hours and begin your fasting again at 7pm in the evening.

During the 16 fasting hours you can drink water and other non-caloric beverages but no solid foods. [63]

There are other methods of fasting ranging from Spontaneous Meal Skipping (skip a meal whenever you want) to the 5 – 2 day fast (where you eat regularly for 5 days but only consume a very small amount of calories on the other two days of each week). [64]

Colored Plates. The Food & Brand Lab at Cornell University reported if there is a high contrast between the color of the food and the color of the plate you are eating from, you will eat less since the color contrast gives your brain the impression you are eating a lot of food. An example would be to eat say a light-colored chicken breast off a dark blue plate rather than a white plate. [65]

Eating the same foods. If you eat the same food every day you may lose weight. You won't be eating junk food if the foods you stick with every day are healthy foods. But, eating the same thing is boring and you might lose interest in eating since you know what to expect.

Before trying an "eat the same food every day diet" check with your health advisor since you might wind up missing important nutrients or vitamins your individual body needs.

Scientists have also reported eating the same thing every day causes less diversity in the type of bacteria in your digestive system. A low diversity of bacteria in your digestive system may lead to obesity. [66]

Spices. Spicy foods can reduce your appetite by increasing your body's norepinephrine and epinephrine levels. The New York Times and other media reported Canadian researchers determined subjects who ate appetizers and added hot sauce to the appetizer ate around 200 less calories than people who did not use hot sauce. [67] Spicy foods increases a person's metabolism which means your body will burn its fuel (food) faster than others. [68]

Meditation. There are several videos on YouTube to help you meditate your cravings away. There are so many we won't reference them, but you may want to search for a suitable meditation tape to help you control cravings and food choices. If you already practice meditation, incorporate your diet, weight loss, etc. into your meditation.

Hypnosis. Like meditation, a hypnotherapist or self-hypnosis may help control your cravings and food choices. There are also many free videos on YouTube to view which guide you to your "special place" so you can deal intelligently with your diet and goals.

Tensing muscles. There is research showing tensing your muscles when you experience a craving or making a food choice will increase your will power. [69] Give tensing muscles a try when you go down the aisles in the grocery or when reading a menu in a restaurant.

Visualization. Courtney Hutchison and the ABC News Medical Unit reported on several scientific studies which showed visualizing yourself eating the food you crave will make you eat less and help you control your cravings. [70] In other words, if you have a craving, pause and picture yourself eating what you crave. It should make you crave it less especially when you know it will keep you from your sincere heartfelt weight range goal.

Acupuncture. Psychological Acupuncture (also called Emotional Freedom Technique – EFT) may be a way for you to successfully deal and control food cravings per an Elements Behavioral Health report on a study by Dr. Peta Stapleton which is very interesting to help you deal with cravings. [71] Acupuncture clinics have been known treat psychological cravings for food and if you are comfortable with acupuncture you may want to check with your local clinic.

Apple Cider Vinegar. Medical News Today recently reported on the success of the Detox Diet which involves Apple Cider Vinegar in the diet. [72] It involves consumption of apple cider vinegar 3 times a day. There may be adverse effects of this diet.

Sleep. WebMD wrote an interesting article on how lack of sleep will make you gain weight. Not getting enough sleep dulls your brain and you wind up making bad decisions on food. The proper amount of sleep (usually at least 7 hours for the average person) will refresh your brain and increase your control and decision making. [73]

Exercise. Fitness Blender had several free exercise videos dedicated to weight loss. [74] New videos are created often on this site and might want to check out the routines for an exercise video which will help you lose weight. If you are experiencing cravings, do a 20-minute exercise video instead of giving in to the craving.

Maintenance After 66 days

Exercise. The American Journal of Clinical Nutrition reported a five-year study on six groups of individuals. These six groups consisted of people who lost weight after dieting and the researchers found one group out of the six maintained their weight within 3 kgs. since they continued their exercise program more than the other groups. [75]

Lose weight slowly. In a recent study, Emily Feig, Ph.D., of the College of Arts and Sciences at Drexel University in Philadelphia, reported she found that those people who initially lost small amounts of weight at the beginning of their diets maintained their weight very well compared to others who lost large amounts of weight when they initially began their diet. [76]

Many people have lost weight and reached their goal but began regaining the weight back after 3 months or so. In the beginning of this book, we discussed the National Weight Loss Registry which keeps track of people who register with them and who have maintained their weight loss (or at least 30 lbs. of it – which is admirable) for at least one year.

There are many others who have succeeded in reaching their goal and maintained their weight. *Common factors*. The NWLR reported many common factors among the 10,000 people who have lost and maintained weight as follows: [77]

Nearly all of them (98%) reported they kept to their diets which was different than the way they originally ate before they went on the diet. That is, they kept to their diets.

Nearly all (94%) of them continued or increased their exercise program and the most common form of exercise was walking.

9 out of 10 registrants averaged exercising at least 1 hour per day.

78% did not miss breakfast and made sure they ate breakfast every day.

75% of them hop on the scale at least once a week.

62% cut their television viewing to less than 10 hours per week. [78]

Habit. Another recent study of 710 people in five different countries determined people who lost weight (and didn't regain weight) did that since they kept to their new eating habits and avoided obesogenic environments (e.g. a food courts in shopping mall). In other words, those who stayed away from sights, sounds and smells of ready food environments became more successful in maintaining their weight. [79]

No teasing. Another recent study found people maintained their weight better after coming off a diet if they continued their dietary eating habits, with a moderate degree of reward eating, plus the absence of psychosocial stress (i.e. they were accepted with their new thinner figures without a lot of attention or stress), combined with strong social support from family and friends. [80]

Personal stories. The National Weight Loss Registry publishes stories as an inspiration to others and to help others keep the weight off. [81]

Some of these stories [82] are the best way to learn how to recognize the reason you want to lose weight and permanently keep the weight off as the years go by.

For example, Emily realized obesity was taking over her life, her thoughts, and her health. She lost over 80 lbs. in four years. She gave up all fried foods and soda pop. She ate more fruits and vegetables and learned to like them very much.

She developed a habit of exercising by doing yoga and walking.

She kept the weight she lost off for four more years by continuing her new eating habits and exercising. She learned to enjoy exercising by doing only the exercising she truly enjoyed.

Another of the NWLR stories is Raul who weighed 344 lbs., was diabetic, had high blood pressure, and had other health issues. Raul and his wife agreed he should see the doctor about bariatric surgery. Prior to having the surgery, the doctor made him take classes on healthy eating. He discovered he was eating far more calories (5,000 to 7,000 calories per day) than he expended. He lost 150 lbs. over the next year by counting calories and enjoying healthy food and is extremely happy with his life.

Pamela had been heavy, or "plump" as she would say, all her life and two things motivated her to try and finally lose weight. First, she hated always having to always shop in the "Plus" section, and second, the engagement of her oldest son. She went to Weight Watchers and learned new things and wound up working for WW and years later she enjoys her new body, her grandchildren, and lots of increased energy.

Jessica originally lost 60 lbs. but didn't intend to lose that much. She gained about 10 lbs. back over 4 years. She lost the 60 lbs. and she exercised by walking and regular gym visits.

Today she eats more than she used to since she expends more calories than she consumes. She does new things too when she eats by enjoying and savoring her food and listening to her body. She loves to use the stepper at the gym and enjoys the feeling of exhaustion after an hour on the stepper. That may seem grueling, but she simply continues her exercising since she enjoys being in her new body.

Another example is Pat, a 63-year-old who had tried many diets over the years and nothing seemed to last. Then she was told her lab test showed she had pre-diabetes. That made her very serious about losing weight and she lost 114 lbs. over the next year and has kept it off for another year and 4 months. She wrote, "I counted carbohydrates and stayed away from refined sugar."

She added she maintained her weight loss by exercising 6-7 times a week, did not eat very low sugar and no refined carbohydrate foods. She used an online support group and found new healthy foods she loves to eat. She wrote she doesn't feel deprived or like she is on a diet and loves her new way of life.

New Developments in Weight Loss

The Fat Switch. April 2017. [83] Research Scientists at Monash University in Australia discovered for the first time how the brain coordinates energy expenditure with eating.

In everyone's body, fat is stored in special cells which change from white (which is the stored fat) to brown (which is fat used for energy) and back again. When you eat your brain signals your body to expend energy and tells your body to turn white fat to brown (energy burning) fat. When you fast, your brain sends signals to store energy which turns your brown fat to white (stored) fat. This process is what makes a person keeps his normal weight.

The researchers found that something goes awry in these processes for obese people. Their fat cells do not turn brown when your body tells it to expend energy. The fat cells stay white when they should be turning brown.

Scientists were puzzled over why this happens. The researchers at Monash University discovered what causes this malfunction and the mechanics involved.

The lead researcher in the project was Professor Tiganis who said, "Our studies have discovered the mechanism that matches energy expenditure with energy intake and this mechanism is defective in obese people. Eventually, we hope to fix this mechanism – or rewire it - so energy will be expended when it should be with resulting weight loss."

Prof. Tiganis advised it may take years of research to fix the mechanism but at least they now know what to fix. Someday it may be that there will be a way we can tell our brain to burn fat in our body without us having to do anything we normally wouldn't do.

Adults need to eat Breakfast. In April 2018, the Mayo Clinic published an article dealing with adults who skip breakfast. They pointed out it was already well established by other scientific studies showing it best for children and teens to always eat breakfast for healthy body, but not much research had been done on Adults.

The Mayo Clinic studied several hundred adults and found a high correlation between skipping breakfast and obesity. They found those adults that skipped breakfast were much more likely to be obese than adults who did not skip breakfast. [84]

The Mayo Clinic recommended to adults to eat breakfast no matter what your age if you want to maintain a healthy weight. [85]

The researchers concluded that regularly consuming breakfast is very important for maintaining a healthy weight at all ages.

Black Tea. A scientific study in the European Journal of Nutrition was published in September, 2018 which found that not only is green tea beneficial to help you lose weight but black tea is also very beneficial to help you lose weight. [86] Black tea is more oxidized than green tea and can be found in the grocery stores and black tea is made by most of the large tea manufacturers like Lipton, Tetley and others.

New findings for strict vegans. Eurekalert announced in 2018 The American Society for Nutrition reported on several studies showing there is more evidence of the other well-known benefits of being on a vegan diet. [87]

The first study was done in the Netherlands of nearly 6,000 subjects which found those that ate more plant-based protein than animal protein had a much lower risk of heart disease in later life. This was because there was a lower accumulation of plaque in the arteries. [88]

Another Brazilian study of 4,500 subjects concluded the same. They found there was clear evidence to show less plaque buildup in later life for those who ate more plant-based protein. [89]

A third study involved South Asians on a strict vegan diet who lived in the US. Those that were on a strict vegan diet had a lower risk of heart disease and diabetes, a better BMI, a smaller waist, lower belly fat, lower cholesterol and lower blood sugar than South Asians living the US who were not on a strict vegan diet and had occasional meat dishes in their diets. [90]

Another 4-year study of over 125,000 adults living the US found those adults whose diets consisted of unrefined grains, fruits, vegetables and nuts didn't have as much weight gain as those adults that ate refined grains such as pasta, fries, white bread, cookies, pastries, ice cream, and cakes. [91]

Another study involved almost 30,000 US adults which found those vegans on strict high-quality vegan diet had a 30% lower mortality rate than vegans who ate a lower quality plant-based protein such as refined grains, pasta, white bread, etc.

They also studied non-vegans and did not find any difference in mortality rates amount meat eaters who ate high-quality animal protein (fish, poultry, etc.) vs. low quality animal proteins (processed meats, lunch meats, etc.). [92]

The Best Diets in the USA. For those who need a strict diet to follow, the US News.com reported in the beginning of 2018, they felt the best diets in the US (in the opinion of their expert dieticians) were: The Dash Diet and the Mediterranean Diet which tied for first place. Third place went to the Flexitarian Diet. In their report, they evaluated and ranked 40 diets. [93]

If you haven't decided on a diet to totally incorporate into your eating habits (and which you will follow for the rest of your life), view the 40 diets in the US News.com report and select one for yourself. Be sure to consider the availability of the food and your daily life schedule. [94]

For those that aren't familiar with the Dash Diet, it is based on fruits, veggies, some low-fat dairy, lean meats, fish, poultry, whole grains, nuts and beans. It is high in fiber and moderate in fat. [95]

The Mediterranean Diet is based on eating fruits and vegetables, fish and other foods. The Mayo

Clinic Staff reports the Mediterranean Diet is very good for heart health. [96]

Remember to always seek the advice of your health professional before going on a diet.

Best to you and we wish you great success with your weight loss journey and to have it become a permanent part of your life so that you will become a more healthier, energized, confident, and better-looking person!

A Food Diary Will Help You Lose

Researchers at the Kaiser Permanente's Center for Health Research have recently shown those who keep a food diary of what they eat each day lose twice (2x) as much weight than those who do not keep a food diary. [97]

You can download a Sample Food Diary from the web like the one offered by the Cleveland Clinic. [98]

We also have provided a very simple food diary for you at the end of this book.

There are numerous free food intake and calorie counter apps which you can carry on your phone or use on your PC and most of them are free:

- My Fitness Pal [99] see their YouTube [100]

- Lose It [101]

- SparkPeople [102]

Simple Food Diary

MONDAY

Date /Time   Food/Drink   How Much

____

____

____

____

____

Notes:

TUESDAY

Date /Time	Food/Drink	How Much

____

____

____

____

____

Notes:

WEDNESDAY

Date /Time   Food/Drink   How Much

____

____

____

____

____

Notes:

THURSDAY

Date /Time   Food/Drink   How Much

____

____

____

____

____

Notes:

FRIDAY

Date /Time   Food/Drink   How Much

____

____

____

____

____

Notes:

SATURDAY

Date /Time   Food/Drink   How Much

____

____

____

____

____

Notes:

SUNDAY

Date /Time   Food/Drink   How Much

____

____

____

____

____

Notes:

About the Authors

TeamGolfwell and Bruce Miller, B.A., J.D. are bestselling authors. Their books have sold thousands of copies including several #1 bestsellers in new releases in sports humor. They live in New Zealand.

Bruce who researched and wrote the major part of this book maintains a healthy weight by not eating any processed food and he regularly exercises (swimming, weight training, golf, exercise videos, etc.). Bruce says, "Forcing myself to wait at least 15 to 20 minutes after eating a moderate meal seems to work best for keeping my weight down."

Contact us at TeamGolfwell@gmail.com. We love to hear from our fans!

www.TeamGolfwell.com

Thank you very much for reading our book and we hope you enjoyed it and you try the techniques for the next 66 days and make healthy eating a lifetime habit for a happier life.

If you liked our book, we would appreciate your leaving a short review on Amazon.

We wish you all the best and great success in changing your life to a healthier and happier you!

We Want to Hear from You

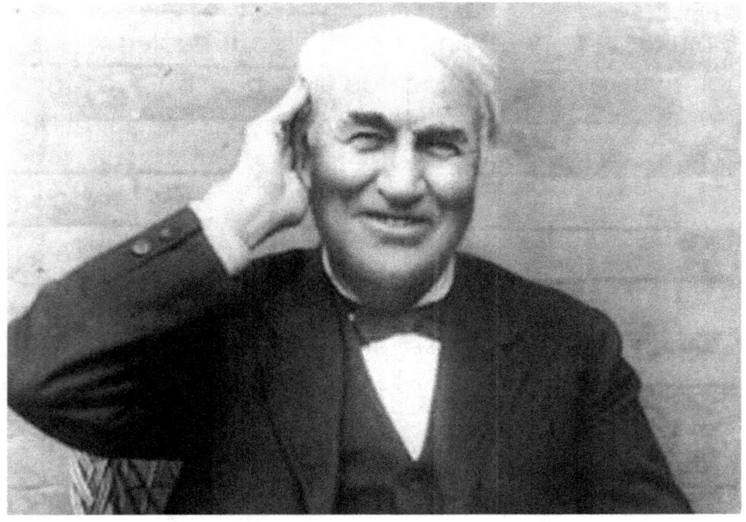

Thomas Edison, image from Creative Commons

"There usually is a way to do things better and there is opportunity when you find it."

- Thomas Edison

We love to hear your thoughts and suggestions on anything and please feel free to contact us at TeamGolfwell@gmail.com.

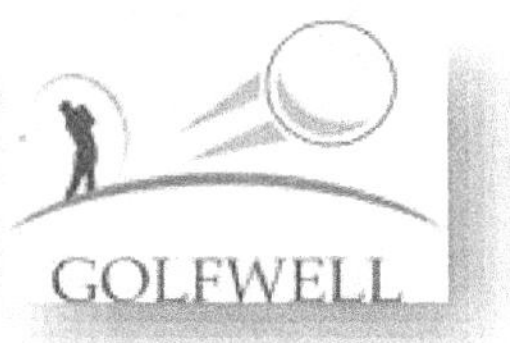

www.TeamGolfwell.com

Team Golfwell's Other Books

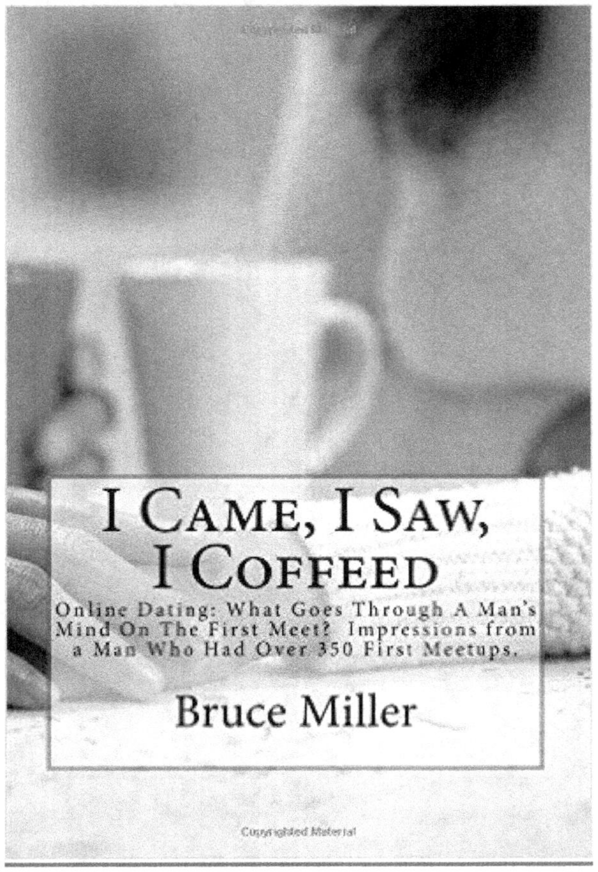

<u>I Came, I Saw, I Coffeed - Online Dating: Why
Didn't He Call Me Back? Impressions from a
Man Who Had Over 350 First Meetups</u>

Team Golfwell's Other Books

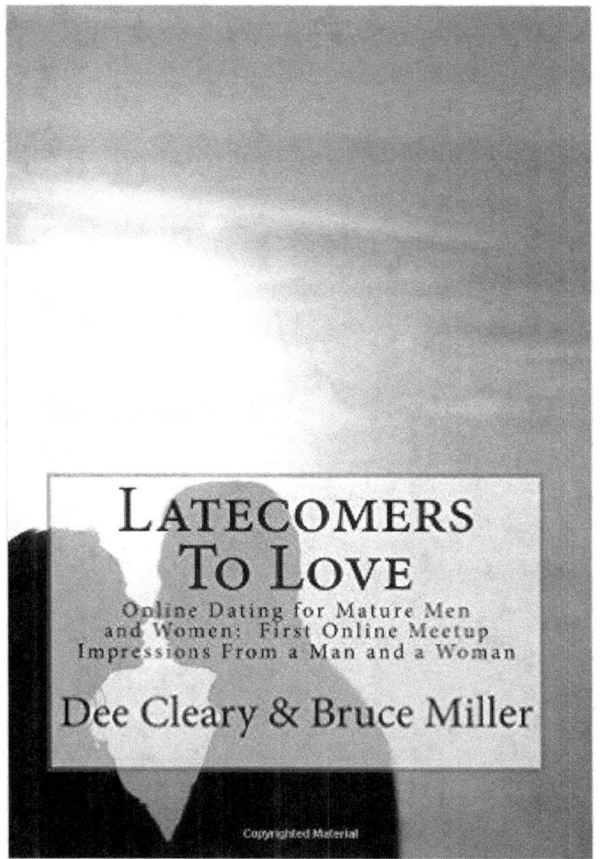

Latecomers to Love: Online Dating for Mature Men and Women: Why Didn't He Call Me Back? Why Didn't She Want a Second Date?

Team Golfwell's Other Books

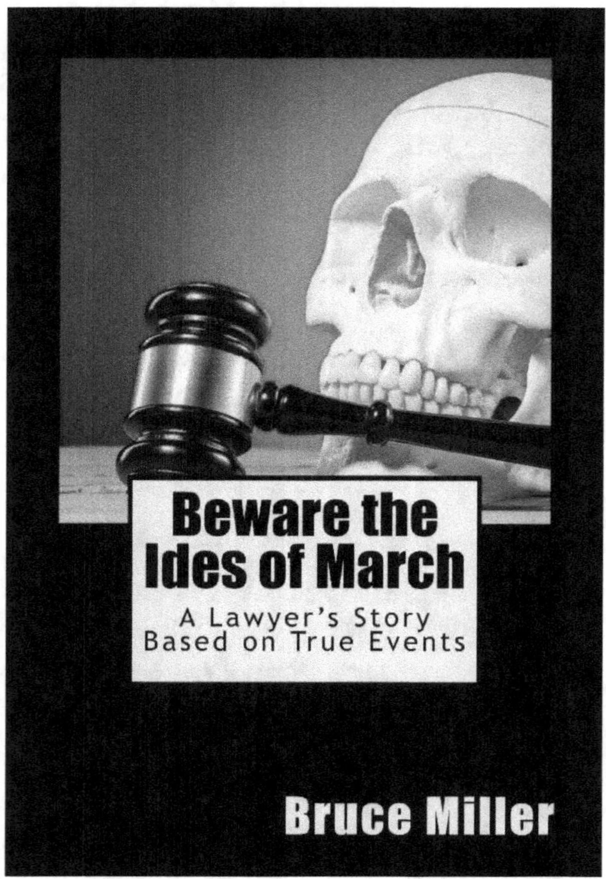

Beware the Ides of March by Bruce Miller a Team Golfwell Member – Based on true events

Team Golfwell's Other Books

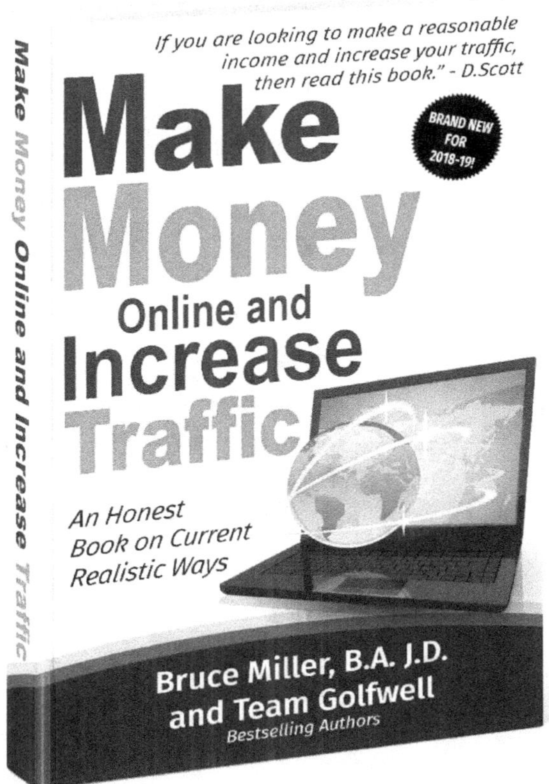

Make Money Online And Increase Traffic

Team Golfwell's Other Books

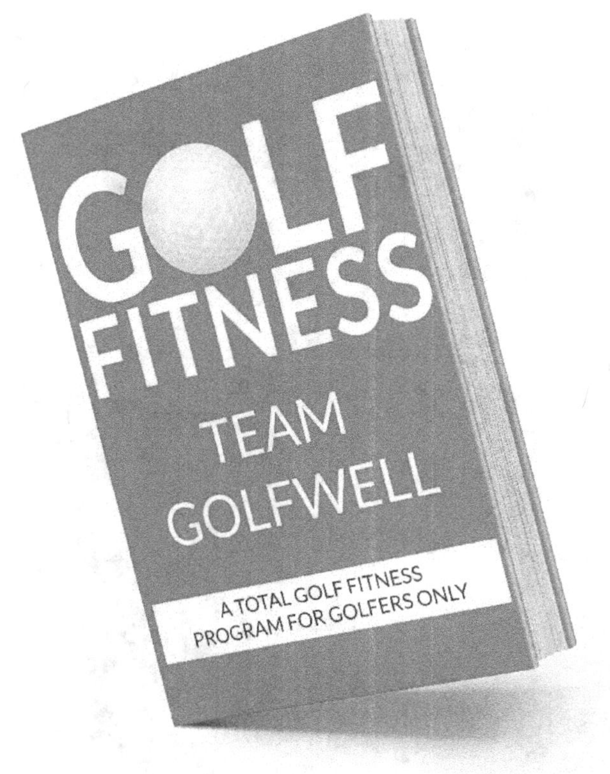

Golf Fitness: An All-Inclusive Golf Fitness Program For Golfers Only

Team Golfwell's Other Books

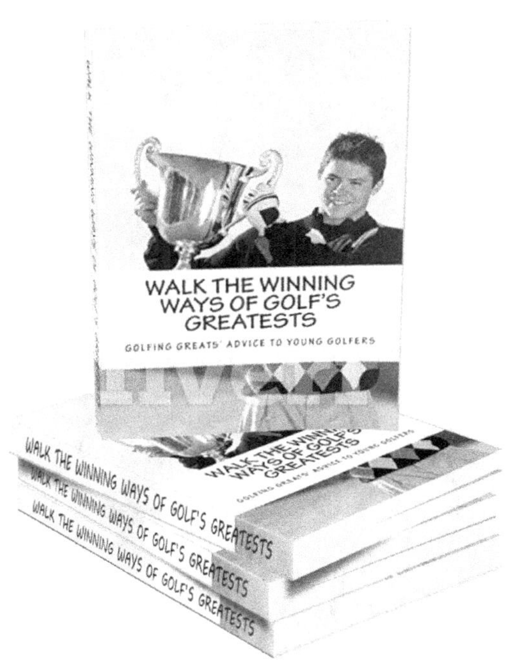

Walk the Winning Ways of Golf's Greatests

For Young Golfers, Junior Golfers, First Tee

Team Golfwell's Other Books

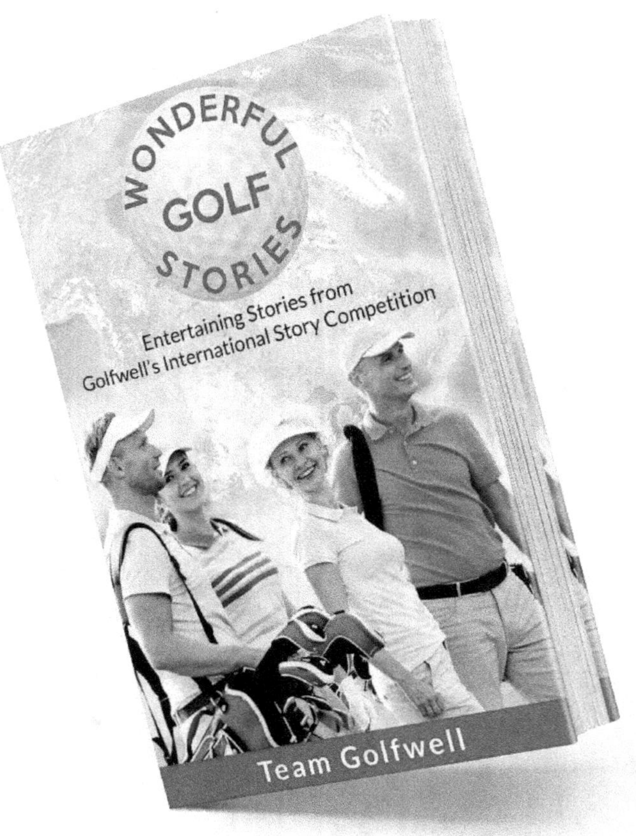

Wonderful Golf Stories: Entertaining Stories from Golfwell's International Story Competition

Team Golfwell's Other Books

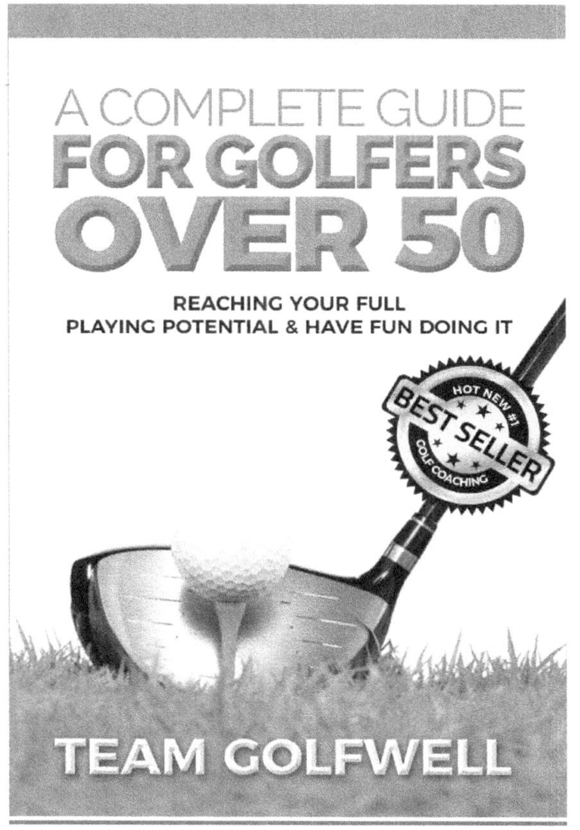

A Complete Guide For Golfers Over 50: Reaching Your Full Playing Potential & Have Fun Doing It. (Over 300 pages)

References

---

[1] British Journal of General Practice,
https://www.ncbi.nlm.nih.gov/pmc/articles/PMC3505409/

[2] Ibid.

[3] Ibid.

[4] The Cleveland Clinic, "The Psychology of Eating",
https://my.clevelandclinic.org/health/articles/10681-the-psychology-of-eating

[5] Ibid.

[6] Susan McQuillan M.S. RDN, Psychology Today,
https://www.psychologytoday.com/us/blog/cravings/200906/change-your-food-attitude

[7] Emma Seppala, "The Happiness Track: How to Apply the Science of Happiness to Accelerate Your Success",
https://www.amazon.com/Happiness-Track-Science-Accelerate-Success-ebook/dp/B00OKJWYB0

[8] The National Weight Loss Registry, http://www.nwcr.ws/

[9] Ibid. http://www.nwcr.ws/

[10] Ibid. http://www.nwcr.ws/

[11] Science Daily,
https://www.sciencedaily.com/releases/2014/04/140428154838.htm

[12] Richard E. Cytowic, M.D, "It Takes Emotion, Not Facts to Change Habits," Psychology Today,

https://www.psychologytoday.com/us/blog/the-fallible-mind/201304/it-takes-emotion-not-facts-change-habit

[13] Richard B. Joelson DSW, LCSW, "Thinking Instead of Doing," Psychology Today https://www.psychologytoday.com/us/blog/moments-matter/201706/thinking-instead-doing

[14] Supra. https://www.sciencedaily.com/releases/2014/04/140428154838.htm

[15] Mayo Clinic Staff, https://www.mayoclinic.org/healthy-lifestyle/weight-loss/in-depth/weight-loss/art-20047752

[16] BCBST.com, https://www.bcbst.com/providers/MPMTools/BMICalculator.shtm

[17] Supra, https://www.sciencealert.com/how-long-it-takes-to-break-a-habit-according-to-science

[18] Scientific Blogging, Science 2.0, https://www.science20.com/news_articles/the_search_for_satiety_neurons_and_how_to_short_circuit_hunger-155142

[19] Ibid. https://www.science20.com/news_articles/the_search_for_satiety_neurons_and_how_to_short_circuit_hunger-155142

[20] Ibid. https://www.science20.com/news_articles/the_search_for_satiety_neurons_and_how_to_short_circuit_hunger-155142

[21] Jonathan Bricker, TEDxRanier, https://www.youtube.com/watch?v=tTb3d5cjSFI

[22] Fitness Blender, https://www.fitnessblender.com

23 Motivate: Daily Motivation,
https://itunes.apple.com/us/app/motivate-daily-
motivation/id1068278823?mt=8

24 Dr. Howard LeWine, M.D., Harvard Health Publishing,
https://www.health.harvard.edu/blog/distracted-eating-may-
add-to-weight-gain-201303296037

25 Ibid.

26 You and Your Hormones,
http://www.yourhormones.info/hormones/peptide-yy/

27 Science Daily,
https://www.sciencedaily.com/news/health_medicine/diet_and
_weight_loss/

28 Physiology and Behavior, "Relationships between human
thirst, hunger, drinking, and feeding",
https://www.ncbi.nlm.nih.gov/pmc/articles/PMC2467458/

29 Ibid.

30 Science Daily,
https://www.sciencedaily.com/releases/2015/08/15082610164
5.htm

31 Mayo Clinic Staff, Snacks: How They Fit Into Your Weight
Loss Plan, https://www.mayoclinic.org/healthy-lifestyle/weight-
loss/in-depth/healthy-diet/art-20046267

32 Harvard Health, https://www.health.harvard.edu/blog/why-
eating-slowly-may-help-you-feel-full-faster-20101019605

33 Prof. Jeff Brunstrom, University of Bristol, "Playing a
computer game during lunch affects fullness, memory for
lunch, and later snack intake,"
https://www.researchgate.net/publication/49673750_Playing

a computer game during lunch affects fullness memory f
or lunch and later snack intake

[34] World Obesity, Online library,
https://onlinelibrary.wiley.com/doi/full/10.1111/j.1467-
789X.2011.00895.x

[35] Ibid.

[36] "Use a Bigger Fork and You'll Eat Less," Catherine
Rampell, The New York Times,
https://economix.blogs.nytimes.com/2011/07/16/use-a-bigger-
fork-and-youll-eat-less/

[37] US National Institute on Health,
https://www.ncbi.nlm.nih.gov/pmc/articles/PMC2864873/

[38] Ibid.

[39] Science Direct,
https://www.sciencedirect.com/science/article/pii/S027153170
5002836

[40] Eric Robinson, Ph.D., Univ. of Liverpool, Institute of
Psychology Health and Society,
https://www.liverpool.ac.uk/psychology-health-and-
society/staff/eric-robinson/publications/

[41] Jeff Brunstrom, Ph.D., Univ. of Bristol, Brunstrom at the
University of Bristol,
http://www.bristol.ac.uk/news/2010/7105.html

[42] Frontiers in Psychology,
https://www.ncbi.nlm.nih.gov/pmc/articles/PMC4630539/

[43] Bioscientifica.com,
https://joe.bioscientifica.com/view/journals/joe/193/2/1930251.
xml

---

[44] Dr. Deborah Cohen, "Candy Out of Sight, Out of Mind", Rand Blog, https://www.rand.org/blog/2017/10/candy-out-of-sight-out-of-mind.html

[45] Ibid.

[46] Kris Gunnars, Healthline, https://www.healthline.com/nutrition/6-proven-ways-to-lose-belly-fat

[47] A Satiety Index of Common Foods, https://www.researchgate.net/publication/15701207_A_Satiety_Index_of_common_foods

[48] Ibid.

[49] Austrian Tribune, http://www.austriantribune.com/informationen/12473-eat-eggs-stay-fit

[50] Ibid.

[51] Ibid.

[52] Ibid.

[53] Science Direct, https://www.sciencedirect.com/science/article/pii/S0031938415300317

[54] Web MD, "Your Hunger Hormones," https://www.webmd.com/diet/features/your-hunger-hormones#1

[55] NCBI, https://www.ncbi.nlm.nih.gov/pmc/articles/PMC5426284/

[56] NCBI, Beneficial effects of green tea: A literature review, https://www.ncbi.nlm.nih.gov/pmc/articles/PMC2855614/

---

[57] Harvard Health Publishing, Harvard Medical School, https://www.health.harvard.edu/blog/artificial-sweeteners-sugar-free-but-at-what-cost-201207165030

[58] Ibid.

[59] The Nutrition Journal of Bio Med Central, NCBI, https://www.ncbi.nlm.nih.gov/pmc/articles/PMC5577766/

[60] Ibid.

[61] Harvard School of Public Health, https://www.hsph.harvard.edu/nutritionsource/healthy-weight/best-diet-quality-counts/

[62] Harvard School of Public Health, Healthy Eating Plate, https://www.hsph.harvard.edu/nutritionsource/healthy-eating-plate/

[63] Leangains.com, https://leangains.com/the-leangains-guide

[64] NCBI-NHI, https://www.ncbi.nlm.nih.gov/pmc/articles/PMC3680567/

[65] Food and Brand Lab, Cornell Univ. https://foodpsychology.cornell.edu/discoveries/color-your-plates-matters

[66] Genome Biology, https://genomebiology.biomedcentral.com/articles/10.1186/s13059-016-1052-7

[67] New York Times, https://www.nytimes.com/2006/11/28/health/nutrition/28real.html

[68] Ibid.

---

[69] Science Daily, https://www.sciencedaily.com/releases/2010/10/101018163110.htm

[70] Courtney Hutchison and the ABC Medical Unit, https://abcnews.go.com/Health/WomensHealth/imagination-diet-visualize-eating-kill-cravings/story?id=12347197

[71] EBH, Dr. Peta Stapleton, https://www.elementsbehavioralhealth.com/news-and-research/psychological-acupuncture-helps-reduce-food-cravings/

[72] Medical News Today, https://www.medicalnewstoday.com/articles/320930.php

[73] WebMD, https://www.webmd.com/diet/sleep-and-weight-loss#1

[74] FitnessBlender, https://www.fitnessblender.com/healthy-living/weight-loss

[75] American Journal of Clinical Nutrition, https://doi.org/10.1093/ajcn/74.5.579

[76] Emily Feig, Ph.D., of the College of Arts and Sciences at Drexel University in Philadelphia, https://onlinelibrary.wiley.com/doi/abs/10.1002/oby.21925

[77] NCBI – NHI, https://www.ncbi.nlm.nih.gov/pmc/articles/PMC4562400/

[78] Ibid.

[79] Taylor & Francis online, https://doi.org/10.1080/17437199.2017.1299583

[80] Obes facts, 2017. https://doi.org/10.1159/000481138

[81] National Weight Loss Registry, Success Stories, http://www.nwcr.ws/stories.htm

[82] Ibid.

[83] Medicine, Nursing and Health Sciences, Monash University, http://www.med.monash.edu.au/biochem/labs/tiganis/publications.html

[84] Ibid.

[85] Ibid.

[86] European Journal of Nutrition, https://link.springer.com/article/10.1007/s00394-017-1542-8

[87] Eurekalert.org, "New research reveals benefits of a vegetarian diet", https://www.eurekalert.org/pub_releases/2018-06/n2-nrr053118.php

[88] Ibid.

[89] Ibid.

[90] Ibid.

[91] Ibid.

[92] Ibid.

[93] US News, https://health.usnews.com/best-diet/best-diets-overall

[94] Ibid.

[95] DashDiet.org, "The Dash Diet Plan", https://dashdiet.org

96 Mayo Clinic Staff, "Mediterranean diet: A heart-healthy eating plan", https://www.mayoclinic.org/healthy-lifestyle/nutrition-and-healthy-eating/in-depth/mediterranean-diet/art-20047801

97 Kaiser Permanente's Center for Health Research, https://research.kpchr.org/News/Press-Releases/Post/343/CHR-Study-Finds-Keeping-Food-Diaries-Doubles-Weight-Loss

98 Cleveland Clinic Sample Food Diary, https://my.clevelandclinic.org/health/drugs/17453-sample-food-diary

99 My Fitness Pal, https://www.myfitnesspal.com/

100 MyFitnessPal YouTube, https://www.youtube.com/watch?v=fu9RKqlmD1Q

101 LoseIt App, https://play.google.com/store/apps/details?id=com.fitnow.loseit&hl=en

102 SparkPeople, https://www.sparkpeople.com/